Carl
Toes First

Carry Me Out Toes First

Martha's Journey

Marilyn Moldowan

Copyright © 2017 Marilyn Moldowan

All rights reserved. No part of this book may be reproduced or transmitted in any form or by any means without written permission of the publisher, except in the case of brief quotations embodied in critical articles and reviews.

This material has been written and published solely for educational purposes. The author and the publisher shall have neither liability nor responsibility to any person or entity with respect to any loss, damage, or injury caused or alleged to be caused directly or indirectly by the information contained in this book.

ISBN: 978-0-978210-82-3

There is a place where we house our bodies,
Where we keep our treasures,
Where we eat, sleep, and love,
Where we raise our families
and welcome our grandchildren.
We take a tiny speck of space,
carve it gently out of the universe,
and we call this place home.

To my mom

Acknowledgments

Some very special people guided me in the process of writing and re-writing this book. Their feedback was honest and to the point. These men and women selflessly gave their time to review the transcript at its various stages and give the needed critiques both in written form and through one-on-one conversations. I am so very grateful that they shared their personal stories. Special thanks to Manford and Ina Colbran, Lynne Herzog, Nicola Roe, Diana Love, and Arlene Dicey.

In my work as a realtor for twenty-six years, I have been witness to hundreds of concerned and loving families helping to move Mom, Dad, Grandma, or Grandpa from their house into a condominium, assisted living, or a nursing home. The sale of the elder's home is one that is always stressful and sometimes, traumatic. This book was inspired by your stories and your experiences, and I am honored to have been able to work with you all and to be a part of a most emotional life event, the senior's decision to sell their home. Please know that I am forever grateful for the trust you have placed in me and it is to you, above all, that I say thank you.

Contents

Introduction	13
Chapter 1	21
Chapter 2	29
Chapter 3	37
Chapter 4	39
Chapter 5	41
Chapter 6	53
Chapter 7	69
Chapter 8	73
Chapter 9	79
Chapter 10	93
Chapter 11	99
Chapter 12	105
Chapter 13	109
About the Author	117

Introduction

To be very clear, the majority of we elders are healthy and well and independent and we do not need your help, thank you very much! We are more than capable of making our own decisions, and anyone who interferes and claims that they know what is best for us, can, quite frankly, go whistle.

~ Anne, age eighty-five,
Calgary, Alberta, Canada

This book tells the real-life story of Martha, a widow, who chose to make the decision to sell her home and purchase a condominium. Her daughter, Debbie, and son, Scott, were supportive of whatever their mom's choices were, and Martha did not want to burden them with her challenges of house maintenance and increasing social isolation. This family had healthy dynamics and it was a pleasure for me to work with them as their real estate agent. It was very clear from Martha's first call to me that the decision to move was Martha's.

At Senior Condo Tours, we get more and more calls from people who are not like Martha: People who request information because they find themselves without any family or spouse and a slowly diminishing number of friends. Sometimes these elders do not want family involved, and we look at how they can surround themselves with resources and professionals, such as a team of their own advocates whose job is to ensure they have sufficient information to make their own choice.

Still, the vast majority of my clients are families. This book was written for the people who have found themselves at a place of needing to take a hard look at the possibility of moving their senior into a place that better meets social, health, and safety requirements. I hear concern in their voices and the desire to do the right thing for their elder family member.

Adult children—often in the fifty-plus or sixty-plus age range themselves—call me about their loved one, who is often a parent in their eighties, with the overwhelming questions of, "Where do we start? What is available? How do we choose?" The different terminology and definitions for very similar living arrangements further compounds the onerous task of sorting through all the housing information.

The good news is that there is an abundance of information available. If the elder chooses to stay at home, there are lawn-care and snow-removal companies, emergency lifeline monitoring, and home nursing for additional peace of mind. Some grocery stores will deliver, and many pharmacies have had delivery service in place for some time.

The bad news is also that there is an abundance of information available. Trying to sift through housing options that are described in magazines, television advertising, and internet searches often results in information that is cloudy and confusing, rather than providing answers that are clear and concise.

The tremendous task of sorting through decades of belonging, possessions, and treasures in the home is overwhelming. The process of repurposing and re-loving belongings often starts when the elder family member no longer resides in the home, but in fact, much of the downsizing can be started with very simple steps months in advance. For example, the concept of *one bag in, two bags out* is easy to adopt. That means for every one bag of groceries or shopping that enters the home, two bags of old papers, donated clothing, or even a small piece of furniture leaves the home. One cabinet or drawer can be emptied every week, and after a year, you can de-clutter a substantial amount from the home following this process.

The questions I cannot help with are, "How do I make him move?" or "How do I make her understand that the house is no longer a good fit?"

This is territory better explored with counselors and therapists, not real estate agents.

The one expression I hear from older people, almost without exception, is the idea of staying put in their home as long as possible, and the desire to be "carried out toes first", hence, the title for this book. If your senior is managing their own finances and personal business, the decision to stay in the home and be "carried out toes first" is their choice. You may not like or agree with people's choices, but that does not necessarily mean that they have become incompetent to make decisions for themselves. You can, however, look at some ways the family can support that choice and to make it easier and safer for the senior to stay at home.

One of my clients flatly told me that if she sold her house, she would lose part of her personality. Maintaining her home gave her purpose and, even though it is increasingly difficult for her to do as she ages, (she is, at the time of this printing, ninety years young), the satisfaction she gets from knowing she can still take care of herself and her house is her reason to get up every morning. It is her reason to live, and it is the lynchpin to her quality of life.

I am well into my third decade of working with seniors and their families. My clients trust that their homes are sold for the best prices possible, in a reasonable amount of time, with minimal inconvenience for the senior and the family. When purchasing a condominium, my clients are shown the complexes that best suit their needs, wants, lifestyles, and price range. We also discuss rental and lease options if purchase is not an option, and I share resources with the family for those choices as well.

The main challenge in writing this book was sorting through my twenty-six years of real estate experience working with hundreds of families and choosing one common theme for the book. Every family is different, the dynamics and personalities vary greatly, and there is no such thing as a one-size-fits-all solution. I based the character Martha on a client whose story is a simple one, one where there are no compelling health issues to accommodate and a family whose prime interest is in making sure Mom was making the right choice for her. The story that is documented in this book is one where Martha, in her eighties, made her own choice to move into a condo.

Carry Me Out Toes First is about a Canadian family and the life events, conversations, and the human experience are all very real. Although I have taken some literary license, Martha's story is based on real life. The characters are real, but the names have been changed.

1

"Hi, Mom!"

Martha was sitting on a little garden stool, leaning forward, pulling up the weeds around the flowers. She straightened up when she heard Debbie's voice, letting her green-gloved hands rest beside her. She looked at her daughter from under the brim of her straw hat, and watched Debbie walk up the sidewalk.

"Hi!" Martha said, with a wave of the oversized green glove.

Martha was always glad when her daughter popped in for a visit. Debbie lived in one of the newer areas of the city, and her commute from the subdivision into the downtown core took her close to Martha's. The visits were often not very long, but Martha appreciated the time spent with Debbie.

This was a sunny Friday afternoon, and Debbie had more time to visit today. The workweek was done.

Martha reached up to Debbie to give her a hug. She patted the skin on Debbie's left arm. She didn't want to leave any dirt on Debbie's clothes. They hugged each other over the deep pink of the peonies.

"What a great day for the flowers. They love the sunshine," Martha said with a lilt in her voice. She reached down to pull a couple smaller weeds and then patted the dirt back down around the base of the stems.

"Mom, you never get tired of the flowers." Debbie smiled and gently touched a pink petal.

"All they need is a little rain." Martha scrunched her face as she glanced up at the sky. There were scattered clouds above, but no sign of the big fluffy ones that would bring the needed moisture.

"It's warm out here," said Martha. "Do you want some iced tea?"

"That sounds good, Mom," she said.

Debbie put out her hand to help Martha stand.

"I'm fine," Martha gently chided and removed the garden gloves, laying them on the sidewalk beside the stool. She placed her hands on her knees and, leaning well forward, generated enough strength in her legs to stand. Martha straightened her back, took a tentative step forward, and once the momentum of walking was assured, carried on toward the front door.

Martha stepped past Debbie and felt her daughter's eyes watch as she made her way down the narrow concrete path at the side of the house to the back door. Martha confidently took the three steps, one at a time, up to the screen door.

Debbie held the screen door open for her mom, and Martha stepped into the back porch. She stopped at the landing inside the house, took off the straw sun hat and hung it on one of the hooks at the back landing. Martha took the handrail and guided herself up two steps into the kitchen. Debbie was just a couple steps behind and gently tried to close the screen door behind her, but the latch was not quite catching the way it usually did. Martha glanced over at Debbie's attempt to secure the door.

"Just leave it, Debbie. That door has not closed properly for a few weeks. I'll get someone in to look at it before winter."

I will just put that on the to-do list, Martha thought to herself. She took a soft breath as she pictured that list in her mind. It was getting longer and longer.

Martha and her daughter continued the visit with chatter about the weather, news events, and updates about the distant family. After washing her hands at the kitchen sink, Martha began to prepare the pitcher of iced tea, and, by sheer habit, glanced up at the clock. There was comfort in seeing the second hand move, halting for just enough time to gather the momentum to move to the next mark on the face with a "tick" sound, and a "tock" sound at rest.

Henry, Martha's husband, had liked the clock up high on the wall, just over the window. Twice a year, he'd reach up over his wife's head, take the clock down, and adjust the time on the clock. His lanky frame would tower over petite Martha, and she'd look up at him, watching this familiar process.

Martha's heart smiled at the memory, one that she relived over and over in the last year. Henry was almost like the Friendly Giant, and once he had adjusted the clock and put it back into place, his upstretched arms would sweep down in one fluid motion to embrace her. Martha remembered how secure and loved she felt in her husband's embrace.

"Mom?"

Martha looked up at Debbie, who had stopped talking in mid-sentence.

"Mom," she said, "you're not even listening to a word I'm saying."

Martha caught Debbie's eyes, which were wide open in mild exasperation.

"I'm sorry. I was just thinking about your dad and his routine for changing the time on the clock," Martha said gently.

Debbie's face softened. "Yeah, that's a nice memory."

"You and Scott would hide behind the corner and ambush us!"

Debbie continued the recollection, "We knew that as soon as Dad hugged you, you would start to giggle. That was our cue to run into the kitchen for a hug, too."

It was a memory that Martha hadn't shared with Debbie in a long time, and now Martha accepted her daughter's hug under the kitchen clock. She knew that her daughter loved her, but the hug just wasn't the same as Henry's hug.

God, how she missed her husband.

2

An hour passed at the kitchen table. Martha and Debbie visited and continued small talk over the pitcher of iced tea, now only with the lemon wedges and a few melting ice cubes left in the last inch of very dilute liquid. A puddle of condensation collected around the base of the pitcher on the red plastic gingham tablecloth. The color of the tablecloth wasn't as vibrant as it used to be, and there were spots where the red color was almost worn away, but it had covered this table for years, and Martha liked it there.

Martha and Henry's conversations had been at this table for fifty years, and she could still see his rough, masculine hands resting on the gingham. His long, relaxed fingers were laced together in front of him, with the thumbs resting down between the palms. He would come in from the garage at lunchtime, wash his hands, and sit down. Martha remembered the easy banter that was so much part of their life. He enjoyed telling her about the way he had fixed minor home repairs. Martha seemed to recall the last repair Henry did was to fix the small leak under the bathroom sink.

Martha's focus came back to the conversation with Debbie. She was lost in the memory of Henry's puttering, and was only half listening to Debbie. Her ears pricked up when she heard Debbie getting ready to leave.

As Debbie moved the chair back from the table, she bumped a small pile of newspapers and magazines with her elbow and they slipped from the plastic tablecloth, to the floor.

"Oops!" laughed Debbie, and reached down to pick them up.

She put the slick magazines back on the table, far away from the edge, and then reached down a second time for the newspapers. There was one newsprint magazine that seemed out of place. Martha watched as Debbie separated this magazine from the pile of paper, held it in her hand, and looked at the cover.

"Shoot", Martha thought, but it was too late. Debbie furrowed her brow together and looked up at her mom.

"What's this, Mom?" she asked gently, and held the magazine up for Martha to see.

"Oh, that," said Martha sheepishly. "It's just something I picked up at the store, you know, from that selection of free magazines."

"But, Mom, it's a magazine of senior apartments . . . ?"

"There are condos in there, too." defended Martha, and then softly, she looked at her daughter. "I'm just looking, Debbie. It just was something that caught my eye."

Debbie was a little taken aback. "Wow, Mom, I thought you told us that you were being 'carried out toes first.' " Debbie teased, raising her eyebrows.

Martha, with a look of feigned indignation, glanced at her daughter and said, "I'm just looking!" After a moment Martha continued. "Your Dad would be so annoyed that I am thinking about renting," explained Martha. "He was all about ownership and having a place where nobody could tell him what to do."

"Yup," laughed Debbie, "that was Dad all right."

Martha noticed concern in her daughter's voice as the conversation picked up again. Martha talked about how she loved the house but it was becoming harder for her to be alone. She really missed Henry. Martha wanted to explain to Debbie that more and more of her friends were either moving away to be closer to their own families or were just not well enough anymore for visits or outings. The house, too, was beginning to look like it needed work.

They briefly chatted back and forth about Henry, the amount of time he spent in the garage with the tools just puttering, and how his home was truly his castle. After Henry retired, he took great pride in keeping the house in tip-top shape. The first thing he did when he noticed even the smallest repair that needed to be done was to put on his shoes and go straight out to the garage to get any tool necessary to fix it up right.

Martha missed that.

As much as Martha enjoyed the flowerbeds in the front yard, Henry enjoyed the lilacs in the backyard. She relived the memory with Debbie about how her dad would sit in their shade for hours, especially during the late spring when the lilacs were blooming in mauve and cream clusters. Martha enjoyed how he brought a sprig or two into the kitchen, and she liked the cream color ones especially, resting on the red gingham.

There was an easy lull in the conversation. The sunglow pouring into the kitchen took on a deeper hue, and Martha was surprised at how the time had gone. She enjoyed the visit with her daughter.

Martha and Debbie stood up from the table and walked slowly from the kitchen toward the door to the backyard. The inside door was open and a light breeze wafted into the living room through the screen door, carrying the scent of the lilacs into the landing. Surprised, Martha looked up at the lilacs, which were now totally green.

They blossomed months ago, she thought, and as soon as she had the thought, the scent disappeared.

She walked Debbie to her car, and stood on the sidewalk as Debbie drove away from the curb.

Martha waved a gentle goodbye.

3

Henry passed away not that long ago. He was sick for a long time and Martha was the caregiver. Last year was a real transition for Martha, but losing her husband after he had been sick for so long was a blessing in disguise. Still, while the burden of taking care of Henry was very difficult, she found the emptiness of the last year even more painful.

It seemed that she saw obituaries of people that she knew more frequently these days. The names were familiar, but there was one especially that shook her.

Frieda's obituary was one that caused Martha to gasp. She decided immediately that she would attend the funeral.

4

Martha closed the door behind her as she stepped back into her home. How she disliked going to funerals. She had seen a few women at Frieda's service who were acquaintances, and polite condolences were quietly shared. Frieda was a friend who Martha had seen less and less often as the years went by: Frieda's health had deteriorated to a point where she did not recognize Martha, and it was far too painful for Martha to continue visiting the nursing home. Martha's memories were of her friend and her visiting other women in the city where they lived, and occasionally playing cards, taking turns at different kitchen tables. The conversations were always lively and the friendships warm.

That seems like a lifetime ago, thought Martha.

Her brow eyebrows rose slightly as she estimated how long ago that had been. Thirty years? Forty? She sighed as she realized how quickly the time had passed. She and Frieda were the last ones left of that group of friends, with the others moving away to live closer to their families or simply passing away.

Martha got lost in her memories for a few minutes and realized she was still standing in the foyer, holding onto her purse. Martha reached over and set it down on the built-in shelf by the closet, took off her jacket, and hung it up. Now only her coats and sweaters greeted her as she opened the closet door; Henry's had been given away to family or donated in the months after he had died.

She shook off the unsettling feeling of being left alone and walked over to the television, turned it on for company, and went to the kitchen to see about supper.

5

Martha found the real estate publication Debbie had teased her about weeks before while cleaning out a stack of newspapers and magazines. Frankly, Martha had forgotten it was even in the house. She sat down as the television chattered away in the background, adjusted her glasses, and turned the newsprint pages one by one.

There was so much information. She looked at the prices and the pictures, and page after page, they all began to look the same. She was trying to understand what she was looking at, but none of it really made any sense to her. She did not even want to think about being in a nursing home. Good Lord, she was way too healthy for that!

"I guess they'll have to carry me out toes first," she said aloud, her lips tightening into a small thin line.

She looked at the page she had just opened to and read the heading out loud:

SENIOR CONDO TOURS

It piqued her interest enough so that she paused and read a little more. There were questions printed on the page that she had asked herself, and she wanted to know more.

> *If you are thinking about a move,*
> *but don't know where to begin . . .*

Martha let out a light "harumph!"

You've got that right! she thought to herself.

> *Maybe you would like more socialization . . .*

Martha's heart skipped a beat. "Yes, that would be nice," she whispered aloud to the television.

The list went on, and then she became curious when she saw that a real estate agent was offering some solutions to these questions. She paused again and looked at the ad. There was a photo of a woman agent who looked a little older than her daughter, but did not look as though she was a senior. The woman looked harmless enough.

Martha read some more.

*Complimentary consultation
in the comfort of your own home . . .*

offered the ad, and:

*Your family is encouraged to be present,
as they may have their own questions.*

"Hmm," said Martha and put the magazine down. She knew that her son and her daughter would support whatever her choice would be, but it just might be time to have a conversation with them. Martha thought some more. She picked up the magazine and opened the page to that list of questions. She folded the upper corner of the page so that she could find it easily again.

Martha walked to the kitchen, took the phone out of the charger, and pressed *auto dial* to connect to Debbie.

Martha was patient as the phone rang four times. Just as she thought she had to leave a message, Debbie picked up the phone.

"Hello," she said.

"Hi," Martha responded.

"Hey, Mom. How are you?"

"I'm fine. But I wanted to run something by you. Do you have a second?" Martha explained a little about the ad that she had just seen and then asked Debbie what she thought.

"Well, it would be good to have more information." Debbie's voice went a little quieter as she said, "Mom, you're really thinking about this, aren't you?"

"I don't plan to move right away, Debbie, maybe in a year or so, but I want to get as much information as I can." Debbie heard her mom continue with a deep breath, ". . . and I don't want to make a mistake."

Debbie hung up the phone and was silent. Her mom surprised her. Wow. Debbie never thought she would see the day when Martha would contemplate a move, but her mom was definitely thinking about it.

The next morning, Martha dialed the phone number from the ad. She was prepared to leave a voice message and was pleasantly surprised when the phone was actually answered.

"Good morning, this is Marilyn," the woman greeted.

"Good morning. I saw your ad and I would like some more information about your 'Senior Condo Tour' service"

"Sure, what would you like to know?" the voice invited.

"Well, I really don't know where to start—" Martha stopped, and then asked, "What is it that you do again?"

The real estate lady went on to clarify. "This service is for people who are in their own homes but are finding that they are wanting, or needing, to make a move at some point. A large part of the challenge many people have had is sorting through all of the information in magazines and advertising, to find out what is really best suited for them."

"Isn't that the truth?" Martha breathed and said, "It is so confusing that I just don't even want to think about it! But your ad says you do consultations. What is that about?"

"We get together for an informal information session at your home, and we have a conversation about what your next home looks like to you."

Martha was still trying to sort it out in her own mind.

"Do you have anyone who would like to be part of this information session?"

"Yes, I have a daughter and a son. That is a good idea. I do want their thoughts, for sure."

"Perfect," Marilyn replied. She continued, "There are three things that may be helpful when we do get together. Do you have a pen and paper? I'll share those with you if you like."

"Yes, I do. Wait a second and I will find a pen that works!" Martha tried four pens that were in her kitchen junk drawer. She was frustrated, thinking how silly it was to keep these things around if they had no ink in them. "Okay, I'm ready."

Martha scribbled on the back of the paper to get the ink flowing, and sat back down at the kitchen table.

"The first thing to understand is what's not working for you in your own home right now. In other words, what is making you think about a move?" Marilyn let some time lapse.

Martha began to think out loud. "Ever since my husband passed away, it's been really quiet around here. My kids are both busy and my friends are disappearing. My television is on for company almost the entire day."

"Wow," Marilyn acknowledged.

Martha was quiet for a second. Why on earth was she divulging her life details to a total stranger? She became uneasy with the disclosure and regained her composure. Martha then shifted the conversation.

"Okay, what is the second thing?" she asked.

"We explore where you have been looking for information: Magazines? Television? Billboards? If you have copies of any publications, it would be great to have them handy."

"I have seen ads on TV, but they go by so fast. I can't read that quickly," said Martha.

"What do you think about keeping a pad of paper and a working pen with you at the television? You might be able to write down a name or phone number when the advertisement is running," Marilyn suggested. "It gives us a starting point."

"Okay, I will get my pile of info together." Martha wrote that down on her notepad. The pen was running out of ink, and Martha asked the real estate agent to hold until she got another one. Martha walked over to the drawer and picked one that looked newer. Martha tried the ink flow on the margin of the paper, and was happy to get a good flow of ink going.

Martha came back to the phone, picked up the receiver and let Marilyn know that she was back on the line.

"One of the first things I should do is throw out all the pens that don't work," Martha joked.

"What would we do without our junk drawers?" Marilyn responded with a light laugh.

Martha poised her pen over the page then asked, "What was the third thing?"

"A city map is the third item that we can use."

Martha was glad this last request wasn't personal. She took a breath as she wrote *city map* on her notepad.

"You mean a real, paper map? I think I have one in the closet," remembered Martha.

"Yes, I think that they are still being printed!" laughed Marilyn, "Please make a mark on the map where your house is."

"Oh? Why is that?" Martha asked.

"We can get an idea of where some apartments and condos are, and see the proximity to shopping and services and stores that are important to you. Right now these places are just addresses in a magazine, but a map will give you so much more information."

After agreeing to call the agent back, Martha hung up the telephone and sat for a minute. She would call the kids, then, and try to organize a time where all three of them could get together with Marilyn.

6

Martha did not get to see her son as often as she saw her daughter. Scott was a sales manager for a car dealership and he seemed to always be in business meetings or traveling to conferences around the country. She received the occasional phone call from him but actual visits took some time and effort to plan. He lived in a city two hours away. Martha found that when she needed him, Scott would always try to arrange to be with his mom. Martha was glad that he took after his father in this way.

Scott arranged the lawn care and snow removal services for the house and for that, Martha was grateful. Even though he could not physically be there, pushing the lawnmower as his father had done, Martha knew that this was Scott's way of taking care of her.

Martha called Scott when she knew he would be at work. The receptionist put Martha through to Scott's line.

"Hi, Mom," said Scott, glancing down at the call display, "How are you?"

"Hello, I'm fine," Martha replied, "How is your day going?"

"Busy as ever, Mom," Scott laughed, then became a little more serious, "What's happening? Did they forget to mow your lawn again last week?"

"No, everything is fine, Scott, the yard looks great," Martha reassured him, "but I want to talk with you about something."

Martha went on to tell Scott about the conversation she had with Debbie, that she was thinking about moving, and that Martha wanted both of her kids to be at the initial meeting with the real estate agent.

"I don't want to make a mistake," explained Martha, "and you and Debbie have experience in the business world. You know what to ask. And I don't want to be forced into signing anything."

Scott agreed and arranged his schedule to be there for his mom.

A few short weeks later, both Debbie and Scott were at their mom's place. They were sitting at the kitchen table when the doorbell rang. Scott glanced up at the kitchen clock above the sink, and noticed that the agent was right on time.

"Good afternoon! I'm Marilyn," said the agent as she reached out to Martha for a handshake.

"Hi, Marilyn, come on in. These are my children Debbie and Scott."

After the introductions, Martha asked the agent whether the living room or the kitchen would be a better place to sit. They settled at the kitchen table and Marilyn took out her notepad and pen, laying them on the red gingham plastic.

"So," Marilyn invited, "you saw my ad in the magazine. What was the one thing that caught your attention? What would you like information about?"

"Well, I saw your ad about 'Senior Condo Tours' and I just want some information and clarification about what is advertised." Martha began. "My kids know that this is my decision but they will support whatever I want to do."

Scott and Debbie both nodded in agreement.

"The trouble is, I don't know what to do!" laughed Martha.

"Wow, yes, the decision to move is huge." Marilyn said, and then continued, "Have you thought about renting an apartment?"

Martha thought for a second and replied, "My husband was always one who believed in ownership, and I like having my own place. I really like this house."

Scott said, "Yes; Dad disliked the idea of putting money into someone else's pocket with rent money that he said was just 'tossed out the window.' There is always the risk of monthly rent being increased or the possibility of the landlord selling the property and putting Mom into the position of looking to move again."

At this point, Martha shuddered, "Oh my Lord, I don't want to be a bag lady. I don't want to be out on the street!" Martha realized that as she lightheartedly spoke the words, she was only half joking.

Both Debbie and Scott piped up and enthusiastically and said that they would never let that happen. Their mom could move in with either one of them at anytime.

"No, that's not what I want, but thanks," Martha smiled and then looked at Marilyn, saying, "I want to do this once and I don't want to make a mistake . . . " Her words trailed off and there was a silence at the table.

"Okay. I understand," the agent softly replied. "What are your thoughts about owning a condominium?"

"Well, there's the thing." said Martha, "I see so much for sale in these magazines, but nothing is available in the areas that I like, and I haven't even heard of most of these areas. The prices don't make any sense to me." Martha then sheepishly admitted, "I would rather not be in a complex that has young families. I have heard of buildings that have an age restriction, but I don't see any of those in these magazines."

"Sure, I get it," said Marilyn. She asked, "Is your map handy? Let's take a look at some of the locations." Scott opened the city map and placed it in the middle of the kitchen table. Martha pointed out some of the complexes in the magazines that looked even remotely interesting, and one by one, the locations were pointed out on the map. This confirmed the concern that many of the buildings offered in the magazines were in the outlying areas of the city and were far away from all of the businesses that she had been going to for decades.

Marilyn gave a partial explanation as to why this was the case.

"Often, the buildings offered in the magazines are new construction, or are newer buildings, and are built where there is land available," she said. "Even though most of my clients want to stay in the same area they live in right now, the reality is that the available land is taken with houses and parks and schools. There is simply nowhere to build. The land is on the edge of the city so that is where the construction happens."

Martha and the kids nodded. "I hadn't thought of that," said Martha.

Marilyn continued, "The builders often use these magazines to advertise and promote their product, and once the building is sold out, they stop advertising. So you only are getting the tip of the iceberg in terms of what is available."

"So, I'm confused," Debbie spoke up. "How do we find out what Mom's other choices are?" She looked at Martha and clarified with her, "You don't want to be on the edge of town—that's far from everything for you."

"Well, I have to tell you, I really like the idea of having something new. When your Dad and I built this house, we were on the edge of town, then, too." Martha's thoughts went to the list of work and upgrades that the house now needed. The house was over fifty years old. Henry would be turning over in his grave if he saw all the work that needed to be done. Her thoughts were stopped by Scott's voice.

"There has to be something closer for Mom. Where are those buildings?"

"I wasn't sure if you needed the information at this point, but I do have information on three good condominium buildings that are pretty close to your house," said Marilyn, and opened her file to produce a sheet of paper. She turned it around on the table so that the family could see the addresses.

She asked that the addresses be referenced on the map, and Scott eagerly took the initiative in finding the locations.

"Mom, this one is just eight blocks away," and he pointed to one address. The family all leaned over the map, and compared all the locations. All three buildings were in locations that were familiar to Martha.

"I didn't see anything advertised about these buildings," she exclaimed, and then said, "This one is closest to me but I had no idea it was an condo complex that I could buy into!" Martha pointed to the location eight blocks away.

"There isn't anything for sale in there right now, but if this looks like a building you'd be interested in, I'll keep an eye out for when a new listing comes on the market, and give you a call to go see it," explained Marilyn, "Does that work for you?"

"Yes, that would be a good idea," agreed Martha, and both Scott and Debbie looked interested in the possibility.

"In the meantime, please feel free to drive past these other complexes and check out the locations. Let me know what you think about them, too" invited Marilyn, "so that I know we're on the right track for what you want."

"None of these are brand new?" Martha clarified.

"Not these," said the agent as she picked up her own printed pages. Her other hand reached over and rested on top of the magazine pile as she continued, "But these magazines list new buildings that we can look at as well."

"Okay," Scott said, "what about those big condo fees? Mom, maybe you should be thinking about just renting."

"Oh, those darn condo fees!" smiled the agent. She continued, "Sometimes a large part of why people choose to remain at home is that exact concern: the fear of condo fees strikes terror into the hearts of seniors everywhere."

Martha, Debbie, and Scott only half smiled. They didn't think it was that funny.

Marilyn took out a sheet of paper with different headings down the right side of the page and blank lines beside the headings. She placed it in the middle of the table. "Here is something you can use to start looking at your current expenses."

"What is this?" asked Martha, and picked up the page.

"It helps you with estimating your actual monthly costs of being in your own home," said Marilyn. "When we do start to look at condos, you will be able to compare the real cost of house ownership with the condo fees. What will more than likely be the case is that the condo fees will actually be less per month than being in your own house."

Martha took her pen, placed her left finger on the printed headings, and began to slowly fill in the blanks to the right.

"Ahem," Scott cleared his throat. "And what about when the fees increase?"

"When your mom finds a building she likes, part of your offer to purchase is a condition that requires full disclosure of all the maintenance that has been done and an estimate of the costs of maintenance to be done in the future." Marilyn went on to explain, "Right now, if the siding on Martha's house needs to be redone, for example, then all the cost is hers. In a condo complex, that cost is divided up between all the owners and there is often money set aside to cover this expense."

"So we get the full financial standing of the complex?" clarified Scott.

"When we write the offer to purchase, yes, absolutely," said Marilyn. "The full information package will ensure that your mom does not get blindsided with an unexpected expense."

The family spent the remainder of the time looking at the map and estimating the time Martha would spend driving to and from her appointments and grocery store. After Marilyn clarified some other questions they had, the family walked the agent to the door, thanked her, and said that they would drive by the locations that she provided.

MARTHA'S LIST

Item	Monthly Cost House	Monthly Cost Condo Fee
Water/sewer	$ _____	included
Heat	$ _____	included
Electricity	$ _____	sometimes
Lawn/snow	$ _____	included
Exterior maintenance	$ _____	included
Insurance	$ _____	included
Security system	$ _____	sometimes
Contingency fund	$ _____	included

(furnace, hot water tank, windows, shingles, etc.)

Value of your time	$ _____	included

(Management of upkeep)

(The above guide is based on an apartment bungalow style condo, without steps and all living on one level. Condo fees vary but an estimate of $400 per month is a good place to start.)

7

The following week, Martha and Scott completed the drive-bys on the three complexes that were closest to Martha's. All three were lovely from the outside and they saw a *For Sale* sign at one of them.

Scott followed his mom into the house and walked over to the kitchen, sitting down at the worn, gingham tablecloth.

"Wow. We didn't expect that," said Scott as he leaned back into the chair. "They all had nice curb appeal and looked well maintained. I didn't even know they were condo buildings!"

"I know, me neither. They had such beautiful flowers on the grounds, too!" Martha replied. "But I still hate paying those condo fees!"

"Where's that page Marilyn gave you, Mom? You know the one to calculate your expenses here in the house?" Martha ruffled through the pile of loose papers and found the single page.

She looked at it then handed it to Scott. "Here," she said brusquely and got up to make some coffee.

Scott reviewed it and said, "Mom, it costs you over a thousand dollars a month to be in this house."

"It's not that much — no way!" Martha argued.

"Look at the numbers, Mom."

Martha's utility bill covered the water, sewer, and heat, and was $300. Electricity was $150, her home insurance was $100 and she was paying the company that took care of the lawn and snow removal another $150 every month.

"That doesn't add up to a thousand bucks, Scott," chided Martha.

"You had to replace the furnace last year and that was three thousand dollars, plus the hot water tank needs replacing soon, Mom. Dad was looking at upgrading the shingles, too, before he got sick, and so that should be done at some point."

Martha was disheartened. She had forgotten about the shingles. Henry had been planning to replace those. How she missed him puttering in the garage and knowing that he was taking care of the leaky faucets, the roof downspouts, and fixing the snowblower for the winter and the lawnmower for the summer. The maintenance was becoming too much for her to handle, even with the handyman service that she had.

"I don't want to talk about that anymore," choked Martha, and she composed herself, blinking back the beginning of tears. Her back was toward her son as she poured the coffee. She shifted the conversation to Scott and his work. Martha needed the diversion.

8

Martha had a restless night. She gently rolled the quilt back and sat up on the edge of the bed, her toes feeling for the slippers that she kept right where she could step into them. There was some dim light coming through the bedroom window, but not enough for her to see. Her wrinkled hand searched for the bedside lamp, and she switched it on.

Standing slowly, Martha straightened her long nightgown and reached for the mint-green flannel housecoat at the end of the bed. She put it on and wrapped herself in the softness. The lamp's warm illumination reached into the hallway and she padded onto the carpet in the hall, making her way down to the kitchen.

The house was in deep silence except for the clock above the kitchen sink that welcomed her with a constant ticktock. There was enough ambient light from the streetlights coming through the kitchen window, so her eyes adjusted easily to the semi-darkness. By habit, she still reached for something a little more solid and touched the fridge door as she walked by on the way to the window over the sink.

There was a heavy snow falling, and she stood at the window overlooking the wonderland that was emerging in the backyard. Huge flakes drifted silently down to kiss her flowerbeds and settle with a thick white in the spreading lilac branches. The serenity was beautiful and she smiled. This is something that she would never get enough of: watching the snow fall. Her hand turned on the cold-water tap and let it run while she took her favourite plastic water glass out of the cupboard. She took good sips of the water and gazed out over the wintry scene again.

Ticktock.

Ticktock.

Ticktock.

Martha remembered all the times in the backyard, Debbie and Scott running around and playing and squealing with laughter while she giggled seeing her children so healthy and happy. She smiled at memories of Henry outside at the BBQ in his man-style BBQ apron and chasing the kids with the sauce-soaked BBQ tongs.

A feeling that Martha had been pushing down for many months began to show up again and she tried to swallow it down. She took another swallow of the water but the emotion would not let go this time.

She thought about her life, and how she and Henry had made such plans for their retirement, travel, and relaxing, and doing it all together.

She was overwhelmed with the thought of moving. She so wished that he were there.

Her tears began to well up.

Her watery gaze caught the lilac branches again, and she blinked at the tears, sending them down the wrinkles of her cheeks. The thick white snow seemed to give her a soft place to fall, and she imagined herself crawling into those open branches, like they were Henry's open arms. She was not able to hold back anymore.

The weight in her throat welled up and burst forth and she cried out the words that were pent up inside her.

"I am so angry," Martha choked and cried.

As she caught her breath between the sobs, she could hear the ticktock of Henry's clock.

"I am so angry at you for leaving me. You left me with all of this to do all on my own."

And then her soul let go with the truth. She screamed at him.

"I am so angry at you for dying on me!"

Martha turned and flung the half-full water glass at the shadow of Henry sitting at the red gingham on the table behind her. The glass bounced twice with sharp pings before it landed and rolled across the linoleum floor.

At the kitchen window that once held so much joy and laughter, Martha and Henry had one more heartbeat together.

This time the view was different.

This time there was no laughter.

This time, she wept.

9

February came way too quickly, and Martha again shook her head at how fast time goes. The television was on but, as Martha prepared her dinner, she was only half listening to the evening news.

Marilyn had recently sent Martha a list of the sales in the neighborhood, and Martha searched for that page again. It was tucked into the folded map. She opened the map at the kitchen table, looked at the addresses on the page, and then looked at the map for the exact location of those houses.

One address caught her off guard. Was that Bill and Mary's house?! She didn't know they were selling! Martha confirmed the address again by looking into her dog-eared, well-worn address book under Mary's last name. Yup, that was their house. *The sale must have happened quickly*, Martha thought to herself, and then slid her finger along the page to look at the sale price beside their address. Martha had no feeling about the number one way or the other; it was the fact that Bill and Mary had moved that had her rattled.

She settled in front of the television with her dinner, and after the news and weather were done, she turned the volume down and picked up the phone. The magazine that Martha used to find Marilyn's service was at the top of her reading pile, open to the agent's ad. She dialed the phone number and left a message.

"Hi, Marilyn, this is Martha. I'm just looking at the page of the home sales near me and, well, I am wondering what my house is worth. You have my phone number. Thanks."

As Martha hung up the phone, she sat and silently asked herself, yet again, if she was doing the right thing.

The agent called back the next morning. Martha picked up on the second ring.

"Hi, Martha. It was good to hear from you last night."

Martha said, "Yeah, I was looking at the page of sales you sent me and I want to know what my house is worth. I'm not selling today, I just want an idea."

"Yes, we can get together anytime this afternoon. Or does tomorrow fit better?"

"I guess I have the time today. I am curious," replied Martha.

Marilyn arrived in the afternoon with a few more pages on the details of the houses that had sold, and gave Martha an estimate of value based on those sales.

Martha looked at the number and said, "That's more than enough to buy a condo, isn't it?"

"Yes, Martha, you have enough," Marilyn confirmed.

"Then I won't be out on the street, " Martha joked, "The kids will be happy that I don't have to move in with them."

Once Marilyn had packed up her briefcase, Martha walked her to the door.

"Thanks, Marilyn," smiled Martha, "I will call you soon."

"You're welcome. It was good to see you again. I'll look forward to your call," and the two women shook hands.

Martha called Debbie and left a message for her daughter about what had happened during the afternoon. Later, Debbie listened to the message, and was a little surprised that her mom had made the call to the agent, but this initiative told her that her mom was closer to a move.

Debbie called Martha back that evening. "You didn't sign anything, did you?" she gently warned.

"No, I didn't," Martha exclaimed. "You know I want to talk to you kids before I do anything. I was just curious about the value of the house and there seems to be more than enough for me to buy something else."

Debbie smiled and asked if Martha had called Scott. "Not yet," said Martha. "I will do that later."

Holy cow, thought Debbie to herself, *Mom is really thinking about moving.*

It wasn't long after that call to Marilyn that Martha thought it was time for another family meeting with the agent. As the four of them sat at the table on Saturday afternoon, Marilyn went over the same information and the sales activity that she had given to Martha, along with the update on new listings in the area.

"So, Mom," asked Scott, "Are you ready to do this? Really?" His voice was soft and respectful to his mother. "You know you don't have to do anything right now."

Martha took a breath and looked at him. "You know what? I am just tired of being by myself, Scott. Your dad took such good care of the house and I can't keep up. The maintenance people that I call are so expensive and the snow removal guy didn't show up again last week. I've had enough. I've been thinking about this for two years and it is time."

Scott and Debbie both looked at their mother and were silent for a moment. Debbie asked the next question, directed toward Marilyn.

"Mom is using money from the sale for a condo, but how do we do this? The money isn't in place until the house is sold, but she needs the money before the house is sold to make that purchase. It seems like a catch-22."

"There are many ways we can look at how that can work," the agent replied. "Do you have your notepad handy? I'd like you to jot down three options."

Martha sat back and just listened to the agent as Scott and Debbie both took out their pens and pads of paper and sat with pens poised.

"One way would be to use savings and investments to pay for the condo." She looked at Martha as she explained, "When your house sells, then the savings is replaced with the sales proceeds. You pay yourself back."

Martha bristled at the thought of touching any of her own savings for the purchase, but she glanced at her children writing that idea down.

"Something else some of my clients have done," continued Marilyn, "is that the family buys the condo."

Scott's head snapped up at this suggestion. "What would be the advantage of that?" he asked with an incredulous tone.

"Well, I have seen it really work well with families when the condo is part of the transition for the adult children if they are looking to move in the future as well. The financial arrangement of who-pays-what is then decided on privately with the family."

Scott's eyebrows went up and he looked at his mom. "How would you like to have me as your landlord?" and he smiled.

"Not on your life am I paying you rent." Martha laughed at Scott. Debbie put her pen down and looked at her mother.

"What about me? That's not a bad idea, Mom. We could work out a deal." Debbie teased as she winked at Martha.

"No. But thanks for the offer." Martha resisted with a lighthearted push on Debbie's shoulder.

"The third way is a more streamlined way to purchase. I would invite you to talk to your banker and have them create a line of credit using your house as the asset. They would lend you money based on your home's value, but you would not use it until you found a condo that you wanted to buy."

"You mean, like using Mom's house as her own bank?" clarified Scott.

"Yes, that's as good a way as any to describe it," said Marilyn.

"I'm confused. How would that be a good thing?" said Debbie, and her mouth twisted into a thoughtful curve.

"The advantage is that when your mom finds a condo that she likes, she can move forward with a purchase, knowing that the money is already in place from this financial arrangement with the bank." Marilyn explained, and looked at Martha. "When we sell your house, then the proceeds from the sales pay the bank back. It's that easy."

"Okay, I get it," Debbie breathed. She looked at her mom. Martha looked overwhelmed. "Mom, what are you thinking?"

"It sounds expensive to do that—borrowing all that money. Lord!" exclaimed Martha.

Scott did a quick calculation on his pad of paper. "Mom, the interest rates are low. This is not a bad thing to consider."

"And *why* would I want to do this?" Martha asked again. Her eyebrows furrowed together.

"It gives you peace of mind knowing that the money is prearranged for your purchase. Selling your house is stressful, and this line of credit can be put in place at a time when there is no immediate pressure to do it. Once we list your house, things can move fairly quickly. It's a piece of your business that can be completed ahead of time," Marilyn said.

Martha took a deep breath and leaned back into the chair. Debbie's hand reached out to her mom and she gently rubbed her mom's arm.

"You okay, Mom?" she asked.

"I'll just sit back and listen right now," Martha replied. This was getting too complicated for her and she was more than happy to let Debbie and Scott ask the agent the financial questions. With every passing minute, Martha found herself withdrawing from the conversation more and more.

Nearly a half-hour had passed with questions and answers among Scott, Debbie, and Marilyn. Martha had enough. She wondered why she even bothered starting this whole mess. Martha was glad to see the agent leave and halfheartedly shook Marilyn's hand. She needed more time to think about this move she thought she wanted.

Debbie reached out to her mom and went to see Martha the next afternoon. She and Scott had talked and agreed one of them should make sure their Mother was okay. They both saw the overwhelmed look in their mother's eyes and how she went silent during the last half of the hour with the agent. They hadn't often seen their mom with that lost look on her face.

"Hey, Mom," she said as she walked into the house. "How are you?"

Martha was watching television, and turned down the volume when her daughter came through the door. "I'm good, Debbie," Martha replied with a heavy breath. "There is so much to think about with all this talk about selling and buying. It's almost easier to just stay put!"

"And be carried out toes first?" Debbie walked over to her mom and gave her a hug.

"Yes! I know why so many people say that. It's just easier." Martha gently shook her head.

"Mom, if you really want to do this, Scott and I have an idea."

Martha listened as her daughter shared the idea with her. Scott and Debbie had agreed to help their mom buy a condominium, and they offered to be their mom's bank. Martha's eyes welled up with tears as she heard Debbie tell her about the conversation that she and her brother had after they left their mother's house the night before. Their conversation with the agent had given them many ideas over and above the three suggestions Marilyn had made, and the kids wanted their mom to know that if she chose to purchase a condominium, that she didn't need to worry about the money.

"There's only one condition, Mom," Debbie grinned.

"Oh, Honey, you two are such great kids!" said Martha as she wiped a tear away from the corner of her eye, put her glasses back on, looked at her daughter and asked with a lopsided smile, "Okay, what's the condition?"

"Well, you'd just pay us back when the house sells."

"That means I don't have to pay you rent?" Martha whooped with laughter.

"No, Mom, you don't have to pay us rent," laughed Debbie, and she enveloped her mom in a warm hug.

10

Martha called Marilyn a couple days later and explained why she had been withdrawn in their earlier meeting.

"I just couldn't handle all the financial detail, Marilyn. It was too much for me to take in and I needed to just back away. But I think I am ready to list the house."

"That's a big step. Please tell me how you came to that decision," Marilyn said.

Martha told her what Scott and Debbie had offered to do and how this simply made the entire move just so easy for her to think about now.

Even though Martha liked the neighborhood where she lived, she found herself drawn to the newer buildings. A couple of phone calls to the agent over the next few days enabled Martha to get enough information about condo living that she was comfortable with the idea of going to look at some condos with Marilyn.

Martha made two things clear to the agent: she did not want anything with stairs, and she wanted a building where there were people her own age. Martha looked forward to having company as much as she looked forward to the idea of no upkeep or maintenance. Marilyn and Martha drove to the areas that were towards the outskirts of the city, and Martha was delighted to see grocery stores, pharmacies, and banks that were the same chains as she was dealing with in her old neighborhood.

"My, my," Martha said, "I had no idea the city has grown so much! These places were open fields when Henry and I built our house."

One building was very much to Martha's liking. It was age-restricted, and the lifestyle there was meant for people who were healthy, retired, and independent. As Martha walked through the apartment condo, she saw that there was lots of light coming through the windows and the floor plan was open and bright. The bedroom was big enough for her furniture and she found that the walk-in closet would probably accommodate most of her clothes.

She stopped as she got to the bathroom, and looked at the walk-in shower.

"Oh, I like that idea." She turned to Marilyn as she spoke, and opened the glass door. It had become more of a challenge for Martha to get in and out of the tub at the house, but she was too embarrassed to talk to the kids about that. Martha had heard horror stories of people who were not able to get out of their tubs once they got in, and she shuddered at having to be there for who knows how long before someone found her.

"There's room for a little bench, too, Martha," Marilyn pointed out. Martha looked at the shower for a long time.

"Yes, that is a good idea," she agreed.

The reality was setting in for Martha that she could possibly be happy somewhere other than her old house. As she stood in the kitchen, her hands rested on the countertop. Martha gazed at the new appliances and at the lever-style kitchen tap. She reached over and turned on the water with just a gentle nudge of her palm. As she shut the water off again, she looked up.

There was room for her dining room table to one side of the main area, and plenty of space for her couch, her television, and the easy chair on the other side.

"There is heated underground parking, too," said Marilyn. "Would you like to see your parking spot?" She smiled at Martha.

Martha looked over at the agent and said, "Hold on, girl, I'm not buying it yet!" and the two of them laughed.

They closed the door to the unit and walked about halfway down the carpeted hallway to the elevator. It was just a quick ride down one level to the parkade, and as Martha stepped out of the elevator, she could not help but think how nice it would be to have her car warm and dry all the time. How she would appreciate not having to clear the snow on her driveway!

They walked past a series of parking stalls; then Marilyn stepped into one of them. "This is the parking spot that goes with your suite — I mean, the suite we just saw," she teased.

Just at that moment they heard the garage door open and a beige four-door sedan slowly coasted down the ramp, turned and drove right past Martha as she stood in the vacant parking stall. Martha eagerly peered into the window of the passing car and saw a woman with short, grey hair who was curiously peering right back at her. The two women smiled at each other and waved.

Martha was getting more and more comfortable with the whole idea. The drive back to Martha's house was quiet, and Marilyn drove, answering Martha's occasional questions.

Marilyn pulled up in front of Martha's house. Martha looked over at her and said, "Let me talk with the kids, Marilyn. I want to make sure that what I'm doing isn't a mistake."

"Of course," Marilyn said, "Good night."

"Good night," Martha responded, and stepped out of the car.

11

Martha did purchase the condominium suite they visited that day, with the stipulation that the condominium financials and documents were in order. It took about a week for the paperwork to be reviewed. With the purchase assured, and a possession date set for six weeks, Martha anticipated being in her new place. Golly, she was getting excited and really looking forward to her next home.

Martha's next step was to sell her house. Both Scott and Debbie were at the kitchen table with their mom when Marilyn explained the listing document to the family. When the contract was signed, the agent slid an envelope over to Martha.

Martha reached in and pulled out two bright orange and black SOLD stickers, and held them in her hand. There was a quizzical expression on her face.

Marilyn looked at Martha, then glanced at Scott and Debbie, who both had their eyes on the stickers.

"Sometimes," explained Marilyn, "the family likes to put these on the *For Sale* sign themselves. Some people take pictures of their parents putting the stickers on the sign when the home is sold. When your house sells, you might want to be the one who posts these."

Martha kept her eyes down as she slowly tucked the stickers back into the envelope. "That's a nice idea. Thank you." Marilyn heard the emotion in Martha's voice.

The *For Sale* real estate sign was on the lawn the next day and, as the agent had promised, there were showings almost immediately. Martha chose to spend the days at Debbie's instead of constantly coming home and going out again when the house was being shown.

On one of the afternoons that her house was being shown to potential buyers, Martha took the time to drive past her new condo building, even though she knew she wasn't moving in for a while. She wanted to see again what was available in the nearby retail mall. In addition to the new clothing and grocery stores, she was pleasantly surprised to see a medical clinic. The choice she had made was beginning to feel more comfortable all the time. Martha went to the bank branch close to her condominium and ordered new cheques with her new address. It was at the pharmacy where she saw a familiar face.

The face was looking back at her.

"Hello." The lady with short grey hair greeted Martha. "You look familiar!"

Martha smiled and said, "Hi, yes, so do you!"

"I'm Clara," the lady smiled and extended her right hand.

"I'm Martha," and smiled back as she shook hands with Clara.

They recognized each other from the parkade, and after a moment of small talk, decided to go to the local doughnut shop just across the street for a coffee. Martha was glad to meet Clara, who had moved into the building just months before. As they chatted, Martha found many similarities between them. Clara, also a widow, was a little older than Martha, and applauded Martha on making the decision.

"I was determined to stay in my house for as long as I could after my husband died. I didn't want to give up and thought that I could take care of all the maintenance. That idea worked until the basement flooded after that storm we had a few years ago." said Clara.

Martha nodded, remembering that very storm. Henry had run outside into the rain and made sure the downspouts were far from the house.

Clara continued, "One of my friends moved into a condo and I visited her one day at her new apartment. I have to tell you, Martha, I was skeptical, but the more I visited my girlfriend, the more I liked the thought of not having to take care of the house anymore."

They finished their coffee with Clara giving Martha gossip about some of the other owners in the building. The building was lively and a new social club had just formed. Martha listened eagerly and found the time with Clara had gone much too quickly. Outside of the coffee shop, they said a warm goodbye and Martha watched Clara walk in the direction of the condominium complex. Martha got into her car and sat for a minute. She was surprised by the feeling of wanting to move into her new home sooner rather than wait until the possession date.

Martha smiled. She knew the purchase wasn't a mistake.

12

About a week after the *For Sale* sign went up, Marilyn gave Martha a call.

"It's been busy around here!" Martha exclaimed, "There are eleven real estate business cards on the coffee table."

"It has been," agreed Marilyn. "One of those agents had a client who wants to buy your house."

"Really!" Martha exclaimed.

"We have an offer, Martha."

Martha's heart skipped a beat.

"Oh, my! What are they offering?" asked Martha.

Marilyn went on to share the details of the offer with Martha. Martha hung up the phone and called her children.

After discussion with Scott and Debbie, Martha called Marilyn back and asked about making some changes to the offer. It wasn't quite what Martha expected and she wasn't sure what to do.

"So what happens now, Martha, is we put forward a counter-offer, which means we go back to the buyer's agent and let them know what works better for you. Nothing is written in stone at this point. What are the changes you want to make?" Martha and Marilyn then talked about the offer and discussed the changes.

"I'd really like one of the kids to be here with me to help me decide what to do," Martha said.

"Perfect," said Marilyn, "I'll be at your house in an hour. Do you think that someone could be with you then?"

"Yes, Debbie lives closer to me than Scott, so she can be here." Martha hung up the phone with Marilyn. One hour, huh? Martha looked up at the clock above the kitchen sink.

Ticktock.

Ticktock.

Ticktock.

13

They all took turns being the designated photographer. Scott and Debbie alternated being at their mom's side as they stood in the front yard beside the real estate sign. The 'SOLD' stickers were on. It was surreal to Martha to think about having someone else in the house. Debbie and Scott were in the first and third grades when Henry built the house. All the trees and lilacs were just planted, not fully grown the way they were now. Her heart felt nostalgic at the memories and yet she knew it was the right choice for her to move.

As luck would have it, the new owners requested possession of the house two weeks after Martha moved into her condo. She was glad for that good buffer of time to move into her new place. Debbie and Scott organized their time so that they could help their mom with both the move into the condo and the emptying of their childhood home. Martha decided to keep much of her favourite furniture, and these pieces fit beautifully into the condo. Taking these large pieces out of the house first made it much easier to distribute the rest of her possessions that were left in the house.

In the kitchen, Martha spent a lot of her time packing smaller boxes. Today, her company was the radio, as the television had already been moved to the condo. The news announcer was her companion as she sorted through the cabinets and drawers. Martha often gazed out at that span of backyard, now beginning to look a little shabby. The snow was melting, and shrubs and patches of lawn started to poke through the white cover.

"Those snow-removal guys haven't shown up again," as she looked at the layer of packed footprints along the garage. Martha realized that she wouldn't need to worry about that for much longer. It was a bittersweet realization.

Neither Martha nor Henry were the particular type of people to hang onto things, but even so, Martha found the task of deciding what to recycle, what to donate, and what to sell, an onerous one. She felt bad calling on Debbie and Scott as often as she did, but the job did get done. Martha left Scott in charge of his dad's possessions and went into the garage only a few times. She was just as glad; she had no idea what most of those gadgets were anyway.

Scott and Debbie both had Martha's blessing to take the items from the house that meant something to them. The garage sale was partly successful: only about half of what they had for sale was sold. Once the family had helped Martha move the things she wanted into her new place, Scott made an unusual suggestion.

"Mom," he said, "there is still a lot of stuff here in the house and garage, and I don't know what you want to do with it. Debbie says she doesn't need these things, either."

Martha looked at the things that, at one time, were meaningful and had value, but she had no use for them anymore. "Scott", she said, "I don't need any of this and I don't have room in the condo even if I did."

"I really hate to take this stuff to the dump. This will sound really weird, but what do you think of this idea?"

Scott described how they could just give things away. Anything from the house that still had some value was carried into the garage. Scott put up a sign on the street Saturday morning that advertised *FREE STUFF* with arrows pointing the way to the garage down the lane. He sat in the backyard, greeting people and watched as they came and went away with armloads of tools, gadgets, and treasures from the house. By noon, the garage was nearly empty.

Scott called his mom at her condo.

"You won't believe it!" he said with delight. "Everything in the garage has found a new home."

Martha gently shook her head and smiled as she hung up the phone with Scott. She was glad someone could use those things. The boxes that had been moved from the house to the condo were nearly empty, with only some bedding and clothes still to be put away. Her television was on as she unpacked the last box of dishes in the kitchen, and saw the old kitchen clock at the top of the stack of plates. Martha took the clock in both hands and looked at it lovingly, then gazed around the kitchen for a place to hang it.

I'll get Scott to put it up for me when he is here, she said to herself and tilted it on edge up against the backsplash so that she could see it. The ceramic of the backsplash seemed to amplify the ticktock sound.

A knock at her door surprised her. It was Clara with the short, grey hair.

"There's a little social gathering down in the rec room. Would you like to come down for a cup of tea?" she invited.

"That would be a good break from unpacking, thanks!" Martha took the key from the hook beside the door and stepped out of her suite, locking the door behind her.

The rec area was a large room with several comfortable chairs, a big-screen television and a wall full of books. Martha noticed a high countertop with bar stools beside the bookcases. A gas-burning fireplace on the far wall had a heavy wood mantel with an elegant oil painting of pink peonies above it. Off to one side of the mantel was a clock enclosed in a glass case, about a foot high, with the brass pendulum swinging silently beneath the clock face.

"What do you take in your tea?" asked Clara.

"Nothing, thank you, just straight up!" smiled Martha. The few people there were talking loudly and seemed to know each other. Strangely, Martha's attention was drawn to a book on a higher shelf, a title that she recognized but never had found time to read.

She was startled by a deep voice behind her.

"Hello."

Martha turned toward the voice and caught his smile.

"Hello" she smiled back.

"My name is Budd."

"My name is Martha."

"Welcome! We all get together once a week." He motioned his arm towards the wall of books. "I noticed that you were looking at our collection."

"Yes," said Martha, "I recognize a title but it's up a little too high for me to reach it."

"Which one?" asked Budd.

Martha shared the title with Budd. As he reached up, Martha noticed his tall, lanky frame. With one sweep of his arm, he took the book off the high shelf and handed it to her.

The clock on the mantel chimed twice.

THE BEGINNING

About the Author

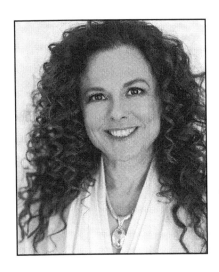

Marilyn Moldowan is a born-and-raised Saskatchewan farm girl. When she moved to the big city of Saskatoon, her first work included being a nurse's aide in a nursing home and helping the music director in a local radio station. She then went into the healthcare field, where she enjoyed years as a home care nurse, assisting clients in their own homes. She later chose a career in real estate, where the skill sets she learned working with seniors and their families while supporting people to stay in their own homes were easily transferred to a successful career. Marilyn excelled at smoothing the life transition and eventual sale of the family home because she treated it with the dignity and respect she learned during her years in healthcare.

The title of this book, *Carry Me Out Toes First*, is a phrase that she heard time and time again from her home care clients as well as from other healthy, independently living, mature adults. The words differed somewhat between people, but that expression of pride and self-reliance was and continues to be a constant for many. Marilyn is currently a senior-in-training at fifty-seven years young.

At the time of this printing, Marilyn has been a real estate agent for over twenty-six years and with ReMax Real Estate (Central) in Calgary, Alberta, Canada, for the last two decades. Her awards include the ReMax Hall of Fame as well as a long-term recognition award from the Calgary Real Estate Board, in recognition of a quarter-century of real estate service. She is a longstanding member of the Better Business Bureau.

Marilyn is looking forward to the next quarter-century of her career as the *Senior Real Estate Specialist*.

Made in the USA
San Bernardino, CA
10 July 2017